This journal has two different sections. The first section is to write down everything you eat and drink for the day. At the bottom of this section, there is a space for summarizing your day and making notes.

You can use this section to write about how you felt that day or the type of day that you had. It's totally up to you. Writing down the type of food that you take is a good way to control your Calorie intake and track your weight loss.

The other section is meant to record your core warm up, upper and lower body workout routines as well as your cool down routines.

Make sure you write down the type of exercise that you do including the amount of sets, repetitions and the time it took you to complete each of them.

Most medical experts recommends you track your exercise routines this way so that you can get first hand information on what you're doing and the kind of result results you're seeing in your fitness and health.

With this, you'll know exactly what you need to do more or work on and also know what's working for you.

That's it. This awesome journal will definitely help you achieve your weight loss goals if you follow it religiously. So go for it, you rock!

DATE:

DAYS	BREAKFAST	LUNCH	DINNER	SNACKS
MONDAY				
Calories				
TUESDAY				
Calories				

WEDNESDAY				
Calories				
THURSDAY				
Calories				
FRIDAY				
Calories				

SATURDAY				
Calories				
SUNDAY				
Calories				

Summary Of My Day

Notes

WARM UP

ACTIVITY	SETS	REPS	TIME	NOTES/SUMMARY

Notes

CORE BODY WORKOUT

EXERCISE	SETS	REPS	TIME	NOTES/SUMMARY

Notes

_____

_____

_____

_____

_____

_____

_____

_____

_____

_____

LOWER BODY WORKOUT

EXERCISE	SETS	REPS	TIME	NOTES/SUMMARY

Notes

_____

_____

_____

_____

_____

_____

_____

_____

_____

_____

COOL DOWN

ACTIVITY	SETS	REPS	TIME	NOTES/SUMMARY

Notes

DATE:

DAYS	BREAKFAST	LUNCH	DINNER	SNACKS
MONDAY				
Calories				
TUESDAY				
Calories				

WEDNESDAY				
Calories				
THURSDAY				
Calories				
FRIDAY				
Calories				

SATURDAY				
Calories				
SUNDAY				
Calories				

Summary Of My Day

Notes

WARM UP				
ACTIVITY	SETS	REPS	TIME	NOTES/SUMMARY

Notes

CORE BODY WORKOUT

EXERCISE	SETS	REPS	TIME	NOTES/SUMMARY

Notes

LOWER BODY WORKOUT

EXERCISE	SETS	REPS	TIME	NOTES/SUMMARY

Notes

COOL DOWN

ACTIVITY	SETS	REPS	TIME	NOTES/SUMMARY

Notes

_____

_____

_____

_____

_____

_____

_____

_____

_____

_____

_____

DATE:				
DAYS	**BREAKFAST**	**LUNCH**	**DINNER**	**SNACKS**
MONDAY				
Calories				
TUESDAY				
Calories				

WEDNESDAY				
Calories				
THURSDAY				
Calories				
FRIDAY				
Calories				

SATURDAY				
Calories				
SUNDAY				
Calories				

Summary Of My Day

Notes

WARM UP

ACTIVITY	SETS	REPS	TIME	NOTES/SUMMARY

Notes

CORE BODY WORKOUT

EXERCISE	SETS	REPS	TIME	NOTES/SUMMARY

Notes

LOWER BODY WORKOUT

EXERCISE	SETS	REPS	TIME	NOTES/SUMMARY

Notes

COOL DOWN				
ACTIVITY	SETS	REPS	TIME	NOTES/SUMMARY

Notes

DATE:

DAYS	BREAKFAST	LUNCH	DINNER	SNACKS
MONDAY				
Calories				
TUESDAY				
Calories				

WEDNESDAY				
Calories				
THURSDAY				
Calories				
FRIDAY				
Calories				

SATURDAY				
Calories				
SUNDAY				
Calories				

Summary Of My Day

Notes

WARM UP

ACTIVITY	SETS	REPS	TIME	NOTES/SUMMARY

Notes

CORE BODY WORKOUT

EXERCISE	SETS	REPS	TIME	NOTES/SUMMARY

Notes

_____

_____

_____

_____

_____

_____

_____

_____

_____

_____

LOWER BODY WORKOUT

EXERCISE	SETS	REPS	TIME	NOTES/SUMMARY

Notes

_____

_____

_____

_____

_____

_____

_____

_____

_____

COOL DOWN

ACTIVITY	SETS	REPS	TIME	NOTES/SUMMARY

Notes

_____

_____

_____

_____

_____

_____

_____

_____

_____

_____

DATE:

DAYS	BREAKFAST	LUNCH	DINNER	SNACKS
MONDAY				
Calories				
TUESDAY				
Calories				

WEDNESDAY				
Calories				
THURSDAY				
Calories				
FRIDAY				
Calories				

SATURDAY				
Calories				
SUNDAY				
Calories				

Summary Of My Day

Notes

WARM UP				
ACTIVITY	SETS	REPS	TIME	NOTES/SUMMARY

Notes

CORE BODY WORKOUT

EXERCISE	SETS	REPS	TIME	NOTES/SUMMARY

Notes

LOWER BODY WORKOUT

EXERCISE	SETS	REPS	TIME	NOTES/SUMMARY

Notes

COOL DOWN

ACTIVITY	SETS	REPS	TIME	NOTES/SUMMARY

Notes

_____

_____

_____

_____

_____

_____

_____

_____

_____

_____

DATE:

DAYS	BREAKFAST	LUNCH	DINNER	SNACKS
MONDAY				
Calories				
TUESDAY				
Calories				

WEDNESDAY				
Calories				
THURSDAY				
Calories				
FRIDAY				
Calories				

SATURDAY				
Calories				
SUNDAY				
Calories				

Summary Of My Day

Notes

WARM UP				
ACTIVITY	SETS	REPS	TIME	NOTES/SUMMARY

Notes

CORE BODY WORKOUT

EXERCISE	SETS	REPS	TIME	NOTES/SUMMARY

Notes

LOWER BODY WORKOUT

EXERCISE	SETS	REPS	TIME	NOTES/SUMMARY

Notes

COOL DOWN

ACTIVITY	SETS	REPS	TIME	NOTES/SUMMARY

Notes

_____

_____

_____

_____

_____

_____

_____

_____

_____

DATE:				
DAYS	**BREAKFAST**	**LUNCH**	**DINNER**	**SNACKS**
MONDAY				
Calories				
TUESDAY				
Calories				

WEDNESDAY				
Calories				
THURSDAY				
Calories				
FRIDAY				
Calories				

SATURDAY				
Calories				
SUNDAY				
Calories				

Summary Of My Day

Notes

WARM UP				
ACTIVITY	SETS	REPS	TIME	NOTES/SUMMARY

Notes

CORE BODY WORKOUT

EXERCISE	SETS	REPS	TIME	NOTES/SUMMARY

Notes

_____

_____

_____

_____

_____

_____

_____

_____

_____

_____

LOWER BODY WORKOUT

EXERCISE	SETS	REPS	TIME	NOTES/SUMMARY

Notes

COOL DOWN

ACTIVITY	SETS	REPS	TIME	NOTES/SUMMARY

Notes

DATE:				
DAYS	BREAKFAST	LUNCH	DINNER	SNACKS
MONDAY				
Calories				
TUESDAY				
Calories				

WEDNESDAY				
Calories				
THURSDAY				
Calories				
FRIDAY				
Calories				

SATURDAY				
Calories				
SUNDAY				
Calories				

Summary Of My Day

Notes

WARM UP

ACTIVITY	SETS	REPS	TIME	NOTES/SUMMARY

Notes

CORE BODY WORKOUT

EXERCISE	SETS	REPS	TIME	NOTES/SUMMARY

Notes

LOWER BODY WORKOUT

EXERCISE	SETS	REPS	TIME	NOTES/SUMMARY

Notes

COOL DOWN

ACTIVITY	SETS	REPS	TIME	NOTES/SUMMARY

Notes

_____

_____

_____

_____

_____

_____

_____

_____

_____

_____

_____

DATE:

DAYS	BREAKFAST	LUNCH	DINNER	SNACKS
MONDAY				
Calories				
TUESDAY				
Calories				

WEDNESDAY				
Calories				
THURSDAY				
Calories				
FRIDAY				
Calories				

SATURDAY				
Calories				
SUNDAY				
Calories				

Summary Of My Day

Notes

WARM UP

ACTIVITY	SETS	REPS	TIME	NOTES/SUMMARY

Notes

_____

_____

_____

_____

_____

_____

_____

_____

_____

_____

_____

CORE BODY WORKOUT

EXERCISE	SETS	REPS	TIME	NOTES/SUMMARY

Notes

_____

_____

_____

_____

_____

_____

_____

_____

_____

LOWER BODY WORKOUT

EXERCISE	SETS	REPS	TIME	NOTES/SUMMARY

Notes

COOL DOWN

ACTIVITY	SETS	REPS	TIME	NOTES/SUMMARY

Notes

DATE:				
DAYS	**BREAKFAST**	**LUNCH**	**DINNER**	**SNACKS**
MONDAY				
Calories				
TUESDAY				
Calories				

WEDNESDAY				
Calories				
THURSDAY				
Calories				
FRIDAY				
Calories				

SATURDAY				
Calories				
SUNDAY				
Calories				

Summary Of My Day

Notes

WARM UP

ACTIVITY	SETS	REPS	TIME	NOTES/SUMMARY

Notes

CORE BODY WORKOUT

EXERCISE	SETS	REPS	TIME	NOTES/SUMMARY

Notes

LOWER BODY WORKOUT

EXERCISE	SETS	REPS	TIME	NOTES/SUMMARY

Notes

COOL DOWN

ACTIVITY	SETS	REPS	TIME	NOTES/SUMMARY

Notes

DATE:				
DAYS	**BREAKFAST**	**LUNCH**	**DINNER**	**SNACKS**
MONDAY				
Calories				
TUESDAY				
Calories				

WEDNESDAY				
Calories				
THURSDAY				
Calories				
FRIDAY				
Calories				

SATURDAY				
Calories				
SUNDAY				
Calories				

Summary Of My Day

Notes

WARM UP

ACTIVITY	SETS	REPS	TIME	NOTES/SUMMARY

Notes

CORE BODY WORKOUT

EXERCISE	SETS	REPS	TIME	NOTES/SUMMARY

Notes

LOWER BODY WORKOUT

EXERCISE	SETS	REPS	TIME	NOTES/SUMMARY

Notes

COOL DOWN

ACTIVITY	SETS	REPS	TIME	NOTES/SUMMARY

Notes

DATE:

DAYS	BREAKFAST	LUNCH	DINNER	SNACKS
MONDAY				
Calories				
TUESDAY				
Calories				

WEDNESDAY				
Calories				
THURSDAY				
Calories				
FRIDAY				
Calories				

SATURDAY				
Calories				
SUNDAY				
Calories				

Summary Of My Day

Notes

WARM UP				
ACTIVITY	SETS	REPS	TIME	NOTES/SUMMARY

Notes

_____

_____

_____

_____

_____

_____

_____

_____

_____

_____

_____

_____

CORE BODY WORKOUT

EXERCISE	SETS	REPS	TIME	NOTES/SUMMARY

Notes

_____

_____

_____

_____

_____

_____

_____

_____

_____

LOWER BODY WORKOUT				
EXERCISE	SETS	REPS	TIME	NOTES/SUMMARY

Notes

COOL DOWN

ACTIVITY	SETS	REPS	TIME	NOTES/SUMMARY

Notes

DATE:				
DAYS	BREAKFAST	LUNCH	DINNER	SNACKS
MONDAY				
Calories				
TUESDAY				
Calories				

WEDNESDAY				
Calories				
THURSDAY				
Calories				
FRIDAY				
Calories				

SATURDAY				
Calories				
SUNDAY				
Calories				

Summary Of My Day

Notes

WARM UP

ACTIVITY	SETS	REPS	TIME	NOTES/SUMMARY

Notes

CORE BODY WORKOUT

EXERCISE	SETS	REPS	TIME	NOTES/SUMMARY

Notes

_____

_____

_____

_____

_____

_____

_____

_____

_____

_____

LOWER BODY WORKOUT

EXERCISE	SETS	REPS	TIME	NOTES/SUMMARY

Notes

_____

_____

_____

_____

_____

_____

_____

_____

_____

COOL DOWN

ACTIVITY	SETS	REPS	TIME	NOTES/SUMMARY

Notes

DATE:				
DAYS	**BREAKFAST**	**LUNCH**	**DINNER**	**SNACKS**
MONDAY				
Calories				
TUESDAY				
Calories				

WEDNESDAY				
Calories				
THURSDAY				
Calories				
FRIDAY				
Calories				

SATURDAY				
Calories				
SUNDAY				
Calories				

Summary Of My Day

Notes

WARM UP

ACTIVITY	SETS	REPS	TIME	NOTES/SUMMARY

Notes

CORE BODY WORKOUT

EXERCISE	SETS	REPS	TIME	NOTES/SUMMARY

Notes

LOWER BODY WORKOUT

EXERCISE	SETS	REPS	TIME	NOTES/SUMMARY

Notes

_____

_____

_____

_____

_____

_____

_____

_____

_____

_____

COOL DOWN

ACTIVITY	SETS	REPS	TIME	NOTES/SUMMARY

Notes

DATE:

DAYS	BREAKFAST	LUNCH	DINNER	SNACKS
MONDAY				
Calories				
TUESDAY				
Calories				

WEDNESDAY				
Calories				
THURSDAY				
Calories				
FRIDAY				
Calories				

SATURDAY				
Calories				
SUNDAY				
Calories				

Summary Of My Day

Notes

WARM UP				
ACTIVITY	SETS	REPS	TIME	NOTES/SUMMARY

Notes

_____

_____

_____

_____

_____

_____

_____

_____

_____

_____

_____

CORE BODY WORKOUT

EXERCISE	SETS	REPS	TIME	NOTES/SUMMARY

Notes

LOWER BODY WORKOUT

EXERCISE	SETS	REPS	TIME	NOTES/SUMMARY

Notes

COOL DOWN

ACTIVITY	SETS	REPS	TIME	NOTES/SUMMARY

Notes

_____

_____

_____

_____

_____

_____

_____

_____

_____

_____

DATE:				
DAYS	**BREAKFAST**	**LUNCH**	**DINNER**	**SNACKS**
MONDAY				
Calories				
TUESDAY				
Calories				

WEDNESDAY				
Calories				
THURSDAY				
Calories				
FRIDAY				
Calories				

SATURDAY				
Calories				
SUNDAY				
Calories				

Summary Of My Day

Notes

WARM UP

ACTIVITY	SETS	REPS	TIME	NOTES/SUMMARY

Notes

CORE BODY WORKOUT

EXERCISE	SETS	REPS	TIME	NOTES/SUMMARY

Notes

_____

_____

_____

_____

_____

_____

_____

_____

_____

_____

LOWER BODY WORKOUT

EXERCISE	SETS	REPS	TIME	NOTES/SUMMARY

Notes

_____

_____

_____

_____

_____

_____

_____

_____

_____

_____

COOL DOWN				
ACTIVITY	SETS	REPS	TIME	NOTES/SUMMARY

Notes

DATE:

DAYS	BREAKFAST	LUNCH	DINNER	SNACKS
MONDAY				
Calories				
TUESDAY				
Calories				

WEDNESDAY				
Calories				
THURSDAY				
Calories				
FRIDAY				
Calories				

SATURDAY				
Calories				
SUNDAY				
Calories				

Summary Of My Day

Notes

WARM UP				
ACTIVITY	**SETS**	**REPS**	**TIME**	**NOTES/SUMMARY**

Notes

CORE BODY WORKOUT

EXERCISE	SETS	REPS	TIME	NOTES/SUMMARY

Notes

LOWER BODY WORKOUT

EXERCISE	SETS	REPS	TIME	NOTES/SUMMARY

Notes

COOL DOWN

ACTIVITY	SETS	REPS	TIME	NOTES/SUMMARY

Notes

Made in the USA
Middletown, DE
21 August 2020